VITALITY BLUEPRINT: YOUR ROADMAP TO A HEART-HEALTHY LIFE

A Holistic Approach to Preventing Heart Disease through Lifestyle, Nutrition, Exercise, and Stress Mastery

Mercy Eunice

DISCLAIMER:

Please keep in mind that the material in this book is intended to be informative only and should not be used as a substitute for professional medical advice, diagnosis, or treatment. If you have any questions about a medical problem, always see a skilled healthcare professional.

Furthermore, the author and publisher disclaim all responsibility for any loss or injury coming from the use of the information included in this book.

TABLE OF CONTENTS

INTRODUCTION

The human heart, a hardworking muscle that constantly pumps lifeblood throughout our bodies, is under attack. Heart disease is a secret pandemic that kills millions of people throughout the world every year. According to the World Health Organization, cardiovascular diseases (CVDs), which include different heart and blood vessel problems, are the leading cause of mortality, accounting for an estimated 17.9 million deaths per year.

This is more than simply a number; it is a personal tragedy with far-reaching effects. Individuals must bear not just the physical and emotional costs of the condition, but also the financial weight of treatments and lost productivity. The loss of loved ones shatters families and puts pressure on healthcare systems.

The threat is considerable, but not insurmountable. Prevention, via a comprehensive strategy, is a formidable weapon against this silent opponent. This book, "Vitality Blueprint: Your Roadmap to a Heart-Healthy Life," promotes this attitude by going beyond a merely medical approach and empowering people to actively engage in their health.

Embracing a Holistic Approach

Traditional medicine is important for controlling cardiac disease, but it should not be the primary emphasis. A holistic approach acknowledges the interdependence of numerous facets of life and their effects on heart health. *This book looks into the four pillars of this strategy and provides practical recommendations on:*

Lifestyle adjustments: Simple but effective adjustments such as prioritizing sleep, eliminating smoking, managing stress, and developing healthy behaviors can have a major influence on your heart health.

Nutrition: Understanding the power of food will teach you how to create a heart-healthy diet rich in fruits, vegetables, whole grains, and lean protein, as well as how to manage the intricacies of fats and salt.

Exercise: Learn about the numerous advantages of moderate-intensity exercise and how to pick an activity you love that fits easily into your lifestyle. We'll also look at the benefits of strength training for general well-being and cardiovascular health.

Stress Management: Chronic stress may be extremely harmful to your heart. This book provides you with effective relaxation practices such as mindfulness, meditation, deep breathing, and yoga to manage stress and build resilience.

"**Vitality Blueprint**" is more than simply a book; it's a tailored guide to a heart-healthy lifestyle. Within its pages, you will go on a voyage of self-discovery, learning about the various forms of heart disease, their risk factors, and your ability to proactively avoid them.

This is not a one-size-fits-all solution. We will look at numerous tactics and allow you to adjust them to your requirements and tastes. *By adopting the concrete strategies and insights provided in this book, you can:*

- Reduce your chance of developing heart disease dramatically.
- Improve your entire physical and mental health.
- Increase your energy level and vigor.
- Live a longer, healthier, and more satisfying life.

The moment to act is now. Let "Vitality Blueprint" be your guide to a vibrant future powered by a strong and healthy heart.

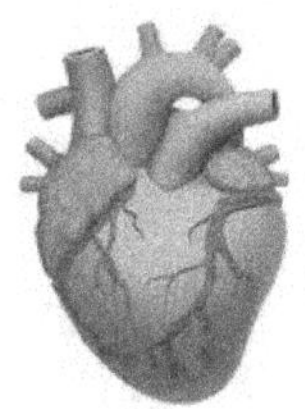

PART 1:

UNDERSTANDING HEART DISEASE

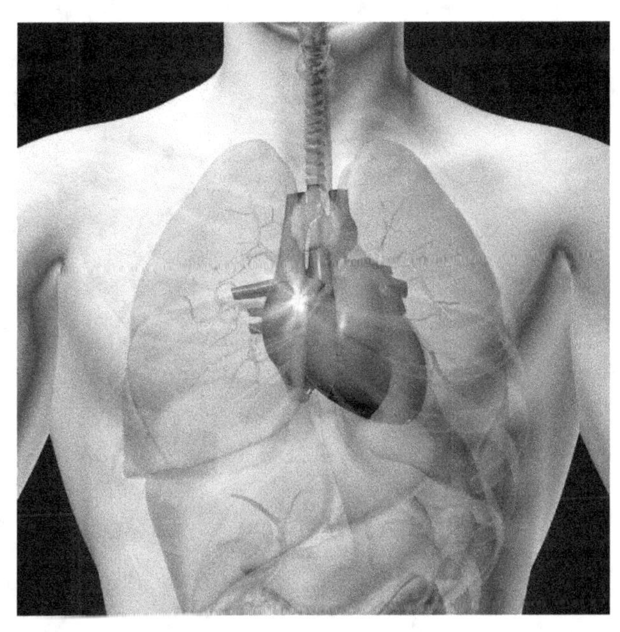

CHAPTER 1: DEMYSTIFYING HEART DISEASE

The human heart, a tireless fighter tasked with pumping life-sustaining blood throughout our bodies, encounters an ever-present foe: heart disease. This umbrella phrase refers to a variety of heart and blood vascular diseases that affect millions of people throughout the world. In this chapter, we'll take a look at the many forms of heart disease, their underlying causes, and the individual risk factors for each.

Different Types of Heart Disease

CORONARY ARTERY DISEASE (CAD): Known as the *"silent thief of hearts,"* CAD occurs when fatty deposits called atheromas form in the coronary arteries, which feed blood to the heart muscle. This deposit narrows the arteries, reducing blood flow and oxygen delivery to the heart. *Over time, this limited blood flow can cause a variety of issues, including:*

Angina is chest pain or discomfort caused by inadequate blood flow to the heart muscle, which is usually initiated by effort and eased by rest.

Myocardial infarction (heart attack) occurs when a blood clot fully plugs a coronary artery, causing permanent damage to the heart muscle.

Sudden cardiac death is a sudden and unexpected loss of consciousness and heartbeat, usually triggered by a massive heart attack that disrupts the heart's electrical rhythm.

ARRHYTHMIAS: These are abnormalities in the heart's normal rhythm that cause it to beat too slowly (bradycardia), too fast (tachycardia), or irregularly. *Different forms of arrhythmias carry varied dangers, ranging from mild to fatal:*

Atrial fibrillation (AFib) occurs when the top chambers of the heart (the atria) beat irregularly, increasing the risk of blood clots and stroke.

Ventricular fibrillation (V-fib) is a chaotic, irregular heartbeat that originates in the ventricles (lower chambers) and can often result in abrupt cardiac death if not treated swiftly.

Premature ventricular contractions (PVCs) are extra heartbeats that originate in the ventricles. They are normally innocuous but can occasionally cause additional arrhythmias.

HEART FAILURE: Despite its name, heart failure does not mean the heart stops completely. Instead, it is a chronic illness in which the heart muscle weakens and loses its capacity to pump blood effectively. *This yields:*

Fluid buildup: As the heart strains to pump, fluid collects in the lungs (congestive heart failure) and other regions of the body, producing shortness of breath, exhaustion, and edema.

Reduced blood flow: The body's organs and tissues do not receive enough blood supply, resulting in symptoms such as exhaustion, weakness, and difficulties exercising.

VALVULAR HEART DISEASE: The heart contains four valves that keep blood flowing in the proper direction inside its chambers. *The disease can impact these valves, leading them to:*

Stenosis is a narrowing that prevents blood passage through the valve.

Regurgitation: A leak that allows blood to flow backward through the valve.

Both stenosis and regurgitation: Depending on the valve and the degree, this can seriously impede blood flow throughout the body.

CONGENITAL HEART DEFECTS: They are structural anomalies that occur at birth and impair the architecture or blood flow pattern of the heart. The kind and degree of the abnormality dictate the specific symptoms and consequences that arise later in life. *Examples include:*

Septal defects are holes in the walls that separate the heart chambers.

Heart valve defects are abnormalities in the structure or function of the heart valves that exist at birth.

Congenital cardiac abnormalities refer to birth defects that affect the general structure of the heart, such as missing or underdeveloped portions.

Causes of Different Types of Heart Disease

While precise reasons may differ, various variables contribute to the development of different forms of heart disease.

Atherosclerosis is a key contributor to illnesses such as coronary artery disease. Over time, cholesterol, fatty substances, and other detritus accumulate on the inner walls of arteries, resulting in atheromas. This process narrows the arteries, reducing blood flow and laying the groundwork for issues such as heart attacks and strokes.

High blood pressure (hypertension): Chronically high blood pressure causes the heart to work harder to pump blood throughout the body, eventually straining and weakening it. This can cause heart failure, stroke, and other cardiovascular issues.

Abnormal Heart Rhythm: A variety of conditions can interrupt the electrical impulses that control the heart's beating, resulting in arrhythmias. Genetics, cardiac disease, electrolyte imbalances, certain drugs, and excessive coffee or alcohol usage are all contributing factors.

Heart valves can be damaged due to several reasons, such as rheumatic fever (a bacterial infection) can induce inflammation and scarring of the valves, resulting in stenosis or regurgitation.

- *Congenital defects:* Some cardiac problems that occur at birth might alter the structure or function of valves.
- *Endocarditis* is an infection of the heart's inner lining and valves that can impair valve function.

- ***Degenerative changes:*** As we age, our heart valves gradually weaken and thicken, increasing the likelihood of stenosis.

Congenital heart defects occur when the heart develops abnormally during fetal development. The exact reason is unknown, although genetics, certain drugs taken by the mother during pregnancy, and environmental exposures may all have a role.

Risk Factors for Different Types of Heart Disease

While certain causes of heart disease are beyond our control, understanding the risk factors linked with each kind allows us to take proactive actions toward prevention.

Coronary Artery Diseases:

- **Age:** Risk rises with age, especially in men over 45 and women over 55.
- **Family history:** Having a close family with CAD greatly increases your risk.
- **High blood pressure:** uncontrolled hypertension is a significant risk factor.
- **High cholesterol:** High LDL ("bad") and low HDL ("good") cholesterol lead to plaque formation.
- **Diabetes:** This illness damages blood vessels and raises the risk of atherosclerosis.
- **Toxins in cigarettes** harm blood vessels and increase plaque development.
- **Obesity** puts a load on the heart and raises risk factors such as high blood pressure and cholesterol.
- **Sedentary lifestyle:** A lack of physical exercise raises the risk of many heart disease risk factors.

- ***Unhealthy diet:*** A diet heavy in saturated and trans fats, salt, and added sweets increases risk factors.
- ***Chronic stress:*** Prolonged stress can elevate blood pressure and have a detrimental influence on several risk factors.

Arrhythmias:

- ***High blood pressure:*** Uncontrolled hypertension can strain the heart and cause arrhythmias.
- ***Thyroid disease:*** An overactive or underactive thyroid can disrupt cardiac rhythm.
- ***Imbalanced minerals*** such as potassium and magnesium can impair electrical impulses.
- ***Certain drugs*** might have negative effects on cardiac rhythm.

- ***Congenital cardiac abnormalities:*** Some congenital defects can predispose people to arrhythmia.
- ***Excess coffee or alcohol*** intake can cause arrhythmias in certain people.

Heart failure:

- ***Coronary artery disease*** is the most prevalent cause, as constricted arteries can damage the heart muscle.
- ***High blood pressure:*** Over time, it can harm and weaken the heart muscles.
- ***Heart valve disease:*** Damaged valves can reduce blood flow and strain on the heart.
- ***Diabetes*** damages blood arteries and raises the risk of heart failure.
- ***Obesity*** increases the burden on the heart while also contributing to other risk factors.

Valvular Heart Disease:

- ***Rheumatic fever*** is a bacterial illness that can damage heart valves.

- ***Congenital cardiac problems:*** Some congenital disorders alter the structure or function of valves.

- ***Endocarditis*** is an infection of the heart's inner lining and valves.

- ***Age:*** As we age, our heart valves gradually weaken and thicken, raising the risk of stenosis.

Congenital Heart Defects:

- ***Family history:*** Having a close family with a congenital heart abnormality marginally raises the chance.

- ***Certain drugs:*** Some medications taken during pregnancy may increase the risk.

- ***Environmental exposures:*** Maternal exposure to certain chemicals or viruses may play an influence (but the data is inconclusive).

Understanding the many forms of heart disease, their causes, and individual risk factors is the first step toward a healthier heart. With this information, you may make educated lifestyle decisions, manage health issues, and collaborate with your healthcare practitioner to create a tailored preventative strategy. In the next chapters, we'll go further into the chain reaction of risk factors unveiling the cascade leading to Heart Disease.

CHAPTER 2: THE DOMINO EFFECT

Consider a row of perfectly balanced dominoes, with each indicating a risk factor for heart disease. A small nudge knocks down the first domino, setting off a chain reaction that results in the last domino collapsing - a catastrophic heart ailment. This chapter explores the domino effect of risk factors, demonstrating how harmless choices and lifestyle behaviors may have a long-term influence on your heart health.

The First Domino: Understanding Atherosclerosis.

The trip frequently begins with atherosclerosis, which is the accumulation of fatty deposits (plaque) in the arteries. This process, like the first domino tipping, initiates a cascade of events that can eventually lead to heart disease. *Here is how it unfolds:*

High cholesterol: Elevated LDL ("bad") cholesterol acts as the first drive. It collects in the artery walls and forms the plaque's core.

Inflammation: The body's natural reaction to LDL causes inflammation in the arterial walls. This adds to plaque accumulation.

Free radical damage: Free radicals, which are unstable chemicals in the body, can damage the arteries' inner lining (endothelium), allowing LDL to build. Factors such as smoking and a poor diet can boost free radical levels.

Calcium deposition: Calcium deposits can accumulate within the plaque, hardening it and narrowing the artery.

The Dominoes Fall: How Risk Factors Accelerate the Chain Reaction

Several risk variables function as extra dominoes, each with the potential to aggravate the cascade and raise the risk of heart disease:

High blood pressure: This presses blood against the weakened and narrowed artery walls, hastening plaque formation and raising the risk of rupture.

Diabetes: This disorder weakens blood vessels and causes inflammation, making them more prone to plaque formation.

Obesity stresses the heart and increases other risk factors such as high blood pressure and cholesterol.

Toxins in cigarettes harm the endothelium, causing plaque development and inflammation.

Sedentary lifestyle: A lack of physical exercise lowers HDL ("good") cholesterol while increasing other risk factors.

Unhealthy diet: A diet heavy in saturated and trans fats, salt, and added sweets is linked to obesity, high blood pressure, and high cholesterol.

Chronic stress can elevate blood pressure, cause inflammation, and have a detrimental influence on other risk factors.

The Final Domino Falls: Possible Outcomes of the Chain Reaction

Left untreated, the domino effect can lead to a variety of cardiac diseases, including:

Coronary artery disease (CAD): As plaque builds up, it narrows the arteries that carry blood to the heart. This can cause angina, a heart attack, or even sudden cardiac death.

Stroke occurs when a blood clot develops within a restricted or blocked artery in the brain, resulting in brain tissue damage and probable long-term impairments.

Peripheral artery disease (PAD) occurs when plaque formation limits blood flow in the arteries that feed the legs, causing discomfort, cramps, and, in extreme cases, tissue death.

The power is in your hands to stop the domino effect and safeguard your heart. Addressing risk factors early on can dramatically lower your risk of getting heart disease and its consequences.

By making educated decisions and making proactive efforts, you may reverse the domino effect and lay the groundwork for a healthy heart and a vigorous life. Remember, while a single domino falling may appear tiny, recognizing the possible ramifications and aggressively responding may make all the difference.

CHAPTER 3: KNOW YOUR NUMBERS

Consider your body to be a complicated mechanism that runs on a continuous basis. Certain "numbers" reveal important information about its interior workings, notably about your heart health. These include blood pressure, cholesterol, blood sugar, and body weight. This chapter digs into the importance of "knowing your statistics," explaining why frequent monitoring is necessary and how they all affect your risk of heart disease.

Blood Pressure

This is the force that shapes your blood vessels. Blood pressure measures the force of blood against the walls of your arteries while your heart beats. *It is expressed as two numerals.*

- ***Systolic pressure (top number):*** Measures the pressure that your heart exerts when it beats.

- ***Diastolic pressure (bottom number):*** Measures the pressure in your heart as it relaxes between beats.

Why It Matters: Chronically raised blood pressure, or hypertension, is a subtle but strong force that damages your arteries and heart over time. *Hypertension stresses the heart muscle, weakens blood vessels, and raises the risk of:*

- ***Heart disease:*** Narrow, weakening arteries restrict blood flow to the heart, paving the way for angina, heart attacks, and heart failure.

- ***Stroke:*** High pressure can burst compromised blood arteries in the brain, causing a stroke.
- ***Kidney disease:*** Hypertension can harm the kidneys' fragile blood arteries, limiting their capacity to function correctly.

Cholesterol Levels

Cholesterol, a fatty molecule generated by the liver and contained in some meals, has an important function in the body but must be controlled. *Here's a breakdown:*

- ***LDL ("bad") cholesterol:*** The major cause of heart disease. High amounts cause plaque development in the arteries.
- ***HDL ("good") cholesterol*** works like a cleaning crew, removing excess cholesterol from the body. High levels of HDL are protective.

- ***Triglycerides:*** A form of fat present in the bloodstream. High amounts, when combined with other risk factors, can contribute to heart disease.

Why It Matters: Your cholesterol profile reflects your cardiovascular risk. High LDL, low HDL, and increased triglycerides promote plaque development and its consequences.

Blood Sugar Levels

They are the fuel that might backfire. Your body's major energy source is glucose, a sugar derived from meals. However, chronically high blood sugar, as seen in diabetes or prediabetes, has subtle effects for your blood vessels and heart.

Why It Matters: *Uncontrolled blood sugar leads to a two-pronged attack:*

- High blood sugar directly affects the lining of blood vessels, causing inflammation and plaque accumulation.

- Chronically high blood sugar levels cause insulin resistance, which occurs when the body fails to respond adequately to a hormone that controls sugar levels. This exacerbates inflammation and increases cardiovascular risk.

Bodyweight

Carrying extra weight, especially obesity, is more than simply a cosmetic issue. *This is a significant risk factor for:*

- ***High blood pressure:*** Excess weight makes your heart work harder to pump blood.
- ***High cholesterol:*** Obesity frequently results in harmful alterations in cholesterol profiles.
- ***Diabetes:*** Being overweight considerably raises the chance of acquiring type 2 diabetes.

How The Numbers Intertwine

While each of these figures is important on its own, they work together to form a complete picture of your heart health. *For example:*

Obesity is frequently associated with high blood pressure, high cholesterol, and diabetes, all of which increase the risk of heart disease.

High cholesterol and blood pressure increase the risk of harm from high blood sugar.

However, "Knowing your numbers" does not cause fear, but rather empowers you to take proactive measures. *Here's why frequent monitoring is important:*

Identifying Hidden Risks: Many people are unaware that they have high blood pressure or cholesterol since they may not experience any apparent symptoms.

Tracking Progress: Monitoring enables you to assess the efficacy of lifestyle changes, drugs, or treatments.

Early detection: Identifying risk factors early enables for appropriate action to avoid or manage consequences.

Understanding your figures is a collaborative process. Your healthcare professional will discuss your goals based on your specific risk factors and medical history. Regular check-ups, which include blood tests and lifestyle conversations, allow you to track your progress and make necessary changes along the way to optimal heart health.

PART 2:

BUILDING THE FOUNDATION – LIFESTYLE MODIFICATIONS

CHAPTER 4: THE POWER OF CHOICE

In the enormous world of health, one reality stands out: you have great control over your heart health. While genetics and certain medical conditions have a part, your daily decisions have a substantial influence on your cardiovascular health. This chapter teaches you to embrace the power of choice by exploring how your lifestyle choices may be the driving force behind a healthier heart.

The Pillars Of Empowerment: Adopting a Heart-Healthy Lifestyle

This empowerment is put into practice through the four pillars of a heart-healthy lifestyle:

1. Prioritizing Health Habits:

Regular physical activity: Aim for at least 150 minutes of moderate-intensity exercise or 75 minutes of vigorous-intensity exercise per week. Even slight improvements in exercise can be beneficial.

Quality sleep: Aim for 7-8 hours of good sleep every night. Inadequate sleep affects hormones and causes inflammation, both of which are risk factors for heart disease.

Stress management: Chronic stress can cause high blood pressure and have a detrimental influence on other risk factors. Meditation, deep breathing, and yoga are all useful techniques.

2. Embracing a Balanced Diet:

Choose entire, unprocessed foods such as fruits, vegetables, whole grains, lean protein, and healthy fats from fish, nuts, and avocados.

Limit saturated and trans fats, which are present in processed meats, fried meals, and baked products, and lead to plaque development.

Moderate sodium intake: Aim for fewer than 2,300 mg of salt each day. This helps control blood pressure.

Limit additional sugars: Sugary beverages, sweets, and processed carbs can all lead to weight gain and other health issues.

3. Quit Smoking (if applicable):

Smoking is a significant risk factor for heart disease and stroke. Quitting smoking at any age will dramatically improve your heart health. Resources and assistance are available to assist you on your journey.

4. Create a Support System:

Surrounding yourself with supportive people who share your desire to live a healthy lifestyle may bring encouragement, inspiration, and accountability.

Empowerment in Action: Making Each Choice Count

The power of choice does not imply spectacular actions or dramatic transformations overnight. It's about actively choosing tiny, sustainable activities that, when added up over time, have a significant influence on your cardiovascular health. *Here are a few examples:*

- Choosing to walk the stairs rather than the elevator.
- Packing a nutritious lunch instead of eating fast food.
- Take a little walk during your lunch break.
- Water will be used instead of sugary beverages.
- Engaging in a calming pastime to relieve tension.

When these seemingly little decisions are made regularly, they have a cumulative impact on your cardiovascular health.

Accepting the power of choice is an empowering journey, not a destination. It entails making deliberate choices, recognizing accomplishments, and learning from losses.

Adopting a heart-healthy lifestyle and actively contributing to your well-being allows you to recover your agency while also improving your heart health. Remember that every decision, no matter how great or little, has the power to affect the future of your heart; choose carefully, healthily, and live a lively life.

CHAPTER 5: SLEEP FOR SUCCESS

Sleep is more than just a passive resting state; it is a period when key biological processes occur that have a substantial influence on cardiovascular health. This chapter goes into the scientific reasons why getting enough, quality sleep is critical for keeping a healthy heart and lowering your risk of heart disease.

What Happens When You Drift Off

Sleep is a complicated dance of physiological changes that are split into phases.

Non-REM sleep consists of three stages: a drop in heart rate and blood pressure, regular breathing, and muscular relaxation. This stage provides physical recovery and metabolic control.

REM sleep is distinguished by fast eye movements, dreaming, and transient muscular paralysis. This stage has important consequences for memory, learning, and emotional regulation.

However, sleep deprivation disrupts the rhythm of heart health. When sleep is cut short or interrupted, your body's finely tuned orchestra falters, causing problems with your heart and blood vessels. *Some of the problems caused are:*

Blood pressure dysregulation: During healthy sleep, blood pressure drops. Chronic sleep deprivation blunts this natural decline, resulting in elevated blood pressure that strains the heart and blood vessels.

Increased inflammation: Sleep deprivation is linked to heightened levels of inflammation in the body. Chronic inflammation contributes significantly to the development of atherosclerosis and cardiovascular disease.

Short sleep duration affects the hormones that govern appetite and satiety (leptin and ghrelin), boosting overeating and weight gain, which contributes to **obesity**, a major risk factor for heart disease.

Insulin resistance: A lack of sleep can lower insulin sensitivity, increasing the likelihood of developing type 2 diabetes, which is a major risk factor for cardiovascular disease.

Sleep deprivation triggers the sympathetic nervous system, **increasing stress hormones** and causing a continuous "fight or flight" state, which strains your heart.

The Sleep and Stroke Connection

Research reveals a concerning link between sleep disorders and stroke risk:

Sleep apnea: This disease, defined by pauses in breathing while sleeping, is significantly associated with high blood pressure and an elevated risk of stroke.

Insomnia: Difficulty getting or staying asleep is related to an increased risk of stroke, presumably due to underlying blood pressure and inflammatory processes.

Short sleep duration: Consistently sleeping fewer than 7 hours each night has been connected to an increased risk of stroke.

The Power of Restorative Sleep

Prioritizing sleep is not a luxury; it is essential for heart health. *Here's how adequate, quality sleep benefits your cardiovascular system:*

Heart rate and blood pressure regulation: During good sleep, these vital indicators normally drop, allowing your heart to relax.

Restorative sleep reduces inflammation by calming inflammatory processes, which promotes cardiovascular health.

Adequate sleep promotes hormonal balance, which helps regulate hunger and maintain a healthy weight.

Improved insulin sensitivity: Adequate sleep improves insulin sensitivity, lowering the risk of diabetes, which is a known risk factor for cardiovascular disease.

Stress reduction: Sleep resets the body's stress system, which helps to regulate stress hormones and blood pressure.

Tips for Sleep Success

To get the heart-healthy advantages of sleep, use these suggestions to improve your sleep environment and bedtime routine:

Consistent sleep schedule: Stick to the same bedtime and wake-up times, especially on weekends.

Dark, chilly, and quiet: Create a sleep-friendly atmosphere with few distractions.

Pre-sleep relaxation: Try relaxing activities like reading, taking a bath, or listening to peaceful music.

Limit screen time: Blue light inhibits melatonin, a hormone that governs sleep, so avoid using electronic devices at least an hour before bedtime.

Seek assistance for sleep disorders: If you suspect sleep apnea, insomnia, or other sleep abnormalities, see a doctor.

Sleep is more than just a break; it is an essential investment in your entire health, particularly the health of your heart. Making sleep a priority and maintaining healthy sleep patterns allows your body to repair, rejuvenate, and protect its cardiovascular system. Prioritize sleep, and your heart will get the benefits of deep, restorative sleep.

CHAPTER 6: BREAKING THE BAD HABITS

Adopting a heart-healthy lifestyle frequently entails not just embracing beneficial behaviors, but also breaking away from negative ones. This chapter digs into three primary factors *"smoking, excessive alcohol consumption, and sedentary lifestyle"* and provides you with the information and solutions you need to conquer them, paving the road for a healthier heart.

Smoking

Smoking is more than just a terrible habit; it is a dangerous addiction with several negative repercussions for your heart and general health. *Here's why breaking the habit is critical:*

Smoking causes damage to the inner lining of blood arteries, leaving them more vulnerable to plaque accumulation, which is a major cause of atherosclerosis and cardiovascular disease.

Smoking raises the chance of blood clots accumulating in the arteries, which can cause a heart attack or stroke.

Reduced oxygen delivery: Smoking lowers the quantity of oxygen delivered by red blood cells, depriving your heart and other organs of essential oxygen.

Smoking causes high blood pressure, which puts additional strain on your heart.

Quitting Smoking

Quitting smoking is the single most important move you can take to enhance your cardiovascular health. *Here are some suggestions to help you along your journey:*

- ***Set a quit date:*** Pick a certain date and adhere to it.

- ***Identify your triggers***: Recognize the events or feelings that make you need cigarettes and devise coping strategies.

- ***Seek help:*** Join a smoking cessation group, speak with a therapist, or see your doctor for tailored advice and support.

- ***Consider using nicotine replacement treatment:*** Nicotine patches, gum, and lozenges can aid with cravings and withdrawal symptoms.

Alcohol

While moderate alcohol drinking may have some stated health benefits, excessive alcohol consumption presents a considerable risk to your heart health.

Excessive alcohol intake can cause high blood pressure, increasing the risk of heart disease and stroke.

Irregular heartbeats: Alcohol can affect your heart's electrical impulses, causing arrhythmias.

Excessive alcohol use can damage the heart muscle over time, reducing its capacity to adequately pump blood.

Excess alcohol use promotes weight growth, increasing the risk of heart disease.

Moderation is crucial during alcohol consumption. *The American Heart Association recommends:*

- ***Men:*** Limit yourself to two drinks each day.
- ***Women:*** Limit yourself to one drink each day.

If you are struggling with alcoholism, get expert treatment to manage your intake and maintain your heart health.

Sedentary lifestyle

A sedentary lifestyle, defined by low physical exercise, is a frequently neglected yet important risk factor for heart disease. *Here's why relocating is important:*

Obesity risk: A lack of physical activity increases weight growth, which is a major risk factor for heart disease.

Insulin resistance: A sedentary lifestyle can cause insulin resistance, which raises the chance of type 2 diabetes, another risk factor for heart disease.

Unhealthy cholesterol levels: Inactivity can lead to an unhealthy cholesterol profile by increasing LDL ("bad") cholesterol and decreasing HDL ("good").

High blood pressure: Sedentary lifestyles are linked to an increased risk of hypertension.

Incorporating Activity into Your Life

Incorporating physical exercise into your daily routine, even in tiny amounts, can offer considerable advantages for your heart health. *Here are some activities that you can incorporate in your routine:*

- Aim to do at least 150 minutes of moderate-intensity activity or 75 minutes of vigorous-intensity exercise per week.

- Break up extended sitting by getting up and moving about every 30 minutes.

- Find hobbies that you enjoy. Choose kinds of exercise that you enjoy and find engaging, since they will be more sustainable over time.

- Begin slowly and progressively increase intensity and duration.

Remember: every step counts! Even little improvements in movement can improve your heart health.

Quitting smoking, limiting alcohol intake, and adopting a more active lifestyle are not simple tasks. However, by recognizing the risks these behaviors represent to your heart and the enormous advantages of change, you can make informed decisions. Use the tactics given, seek assistance when required, and celebrate your accomplishments along the way. Remember that every day you live a healthy lifestyle is a step closer to a stronger, healthier heart.

CHAPTER 7: CULTIVATING HEALTHY HABITS

Your quest for a healthier heart goes beyond merely avoiding dangerous habits. It's about deliberately creating beneficial lifestyle habits that serve as the foundation for a robust, resilient cardiovascular system. This chapter delves into three critical areas: *relaxation methods, social relationships, and keeping a healthy weight*, emphasizing their importance and providing practical solutions for implementing them into your life.

The Art of Relaxation

Chronic stress is more than just a mental burden; it may have serious consequences for your physical health, particularly your heart. *Here's why adding relaxation methods into your everyday routine is important:*

Stress and inflammation: Chronic stress causes the release of hormones such as cortisol, which contributes to inflammation, a critical factor in the development of atherosclerosis.

High blood pressure: Stress can cause a brief increase in blood pressure, which, if prolonged, can damage blood vessels and raise the risk of heart disease.

Poor behaviors: Stress can lead to poor coping techniques such as binge eating or smoking, which can jeopardize heart health.

Nevertheless, you can explore and use the following ways to cultivate calm and successfully manage stress:

Mindfulness meditation is focusing on the present moment and observing your thoughts and feelings without judgment.

Deep breathing exercises: Slow, regulated breaths trigger the body's relaxation response, which lowers heart rate and blood pressure.

Progressive muscle relaxation involves gradually tensing and relaxing distinct muscle groups, creating both physical and mental calm.

Yoga and Tai Chi are mind-body activities that incorporate mild movement, breathing exercises, and meditation to promote relaxation and reduce stress.

Engage in pastimes that you enjoy: Engaging in enjoyable activities can help you take your mind off tension and relax.

The Power of Connection

Strong social relationships are more than simply a source of happiness; they also have a big influence on your physical and mental health, as well as your heart. *Here's why maintaining social relationships is critical:*

Reduced stress and loneliness: Strong social ties create a sense of belonging and support, which can mitigate the negative impacts of stress and loneliness, both of which are risk factors for cardiovascular disease.

Motivation and accountability: Having a support system may help you make healthy choices and hold yourself responsible for your objectives.

Shared experience and knowledge: Connecting with others who are having similar issues or have successfully embraced healthy behaviors may give vital insights and motivation.

Strategies to Build Your Social Circle

Here are some techniques to improve your social relationships and create a support network:

- Spend quality time with loved ones by prioritizing meaningful connections with family and friends.
- Join a club or group to connect with others who share your interests and hobbies.
- Volunteer in your community: Helping others is a gratifying way to build relationships and a feeling of purpose.

- Seek professional help: If you are experiencing social isolation or loneliness, you might consider seeing a therapist or counselor.

Striving for a Healthy Weight

Maintaining a healthy weight is critical for your entire health, particularly your heart. *Here's why.*

Excess weight: Obesity is a major risk factor for cardiovascular disease. It puts additional strain on the heart, contributing to excessive blood pressure, insulin resistance, and harmful cholesterol levels.

Maintaining a healthy weight eases the strain on your heart, improves blood pressure and cholesterol levels, and lowers your chance of developing type 2 diabetes, all of which contribute to a healthier cardiovascular system.

Finding Your Healthy Weight

Achieving and maintaining a healthy weight is an individual journey. *Here are some sustainable solutions:*

- *A healthy diet* should include whole, unprocessed foods, fruits, vegetables, and whole grains.
- *Incorporate physical activity:* Regular exercise helps with weight management, cardiovascular health, and mood.
- *Mindful eating* involves paying attention to hunger and fullness cues to avoid overeating.
- *Seek expert assistance:* Consult a certified dietician or a healthcare professional for specific advice on obtaining and maintaining a healthy weight.

Remember that developing healthy behaviors is a process, not a destination. Celebrate your accomplishments, be fair to yourself during failures, and concentrate on progress rather than perfection. By implementing relaxation techniques, cultivating social relationships, and aiming for a healthy weight, you are actively laying the groundwork for a stronger, healthier heart and a happier life.

PART 3:

FUELING YOUR HEART - NUTRITION

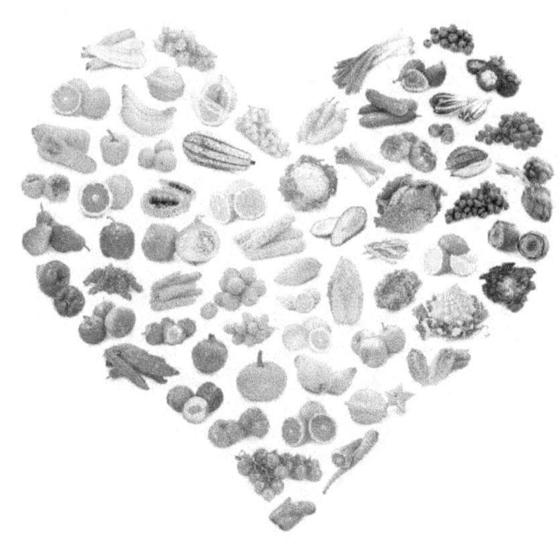

CHAPTER 8: BUILDING BLOCKS OF A HEALTHY DIET

Your heart is a strong engine, and like any engine, it needs the optimum fuel to work properly. This chapter goes into the fundamentals of a heart-healthy diet, highlighting the value of fruits, vegetables, whole grains, and lean protein. Understanding these nutritional-building elements allows you to make educated decisions that fuel your body while also protecting your heart and general health.

Core Principles of a Heart-Healthy Diet

Focus on entire, unprocessed foods, such as whole grains, fruits, vegetables, legumes, nuts, seeds, and lean protein. These foods are high in critical nutrients, antioxidants, and fiber, all of which promote heart health.

Limit saturated and trans fats: These fats, present in processed meats, fried meals, and baked products, lead to plaque accumulation in arteries, raising the risk of heart disease.

Choose Healthy Fats: Fatty fish, avocados, olive oil, almonds, and seeds provide unsaturated fats, which are good for your heart. They can help reduce LDL ("bad") cholesterol while increasing HDL ("good") cholesterol.

Moderate sodium intake: Aim for fewer than 2,300 mg of salt each day. Reducing salt consumption helps regulate blood pressure, which is a major risk factor for heart disease.

Limit added sugars: Sugary beverages, sweets, and refined carbs can cause weight gain, high cholesterol, and an increased risk of type 2 diabetes, all of which are bad for your heart.

Read the food labels: When choosing foods, consider portion sizes, saturated and trans fat levels, salt content, and added sugar content.

Fruits and Vegetables

Fruit and vegetables are essential components of a heart-healthy diet. *Here's how:*

Rich in vitamins, minerals, and antioxidants: These micronutrients are essential for many biological processes and can help protect against chronic illnesses such as heart disease.

High fiber content: Fiber regulates cholesterol levels, increases satiety, and improves digestion, all of which contribute to a healthy weight and general well-being.

Different fruits and vegetables have varied advantages. Berries are high in antioxidants, leafy greens are high in vitamins and minerals, and cruciferous veggies such as broccoli and cauliflower may provide further protection against heart disease.

Aim for at least 5 servings of fruits and vegetables every day, including a range of colors and varieties to optimize the benefits.

Whole Grains and Lean Protein.

Whole grains give continuous energy and critical minerals for the heart.

- **Fiber-rich:** Like fruits and vegetables, whole grains such as brown rice, quinoa, oats, and whole-wheat bread help manage cholesterol, increase satiety, and contribute to a healthy weight.

- **Whole grains** are high in B vitamins, magnesium, and other critical elements that help with a variety of biological processes, including cardiovascular health.

Choose lean protein sources to fuel your body and control your weight:

- **Fish:** Fatty fish such as salmon, tuna, and mackerel contain omega-3 fatty acids, which have been demonstrated to decrease inflammation and lessen the risk of heart disease.
- **Poultry:** Choose skinless chicken or turkey breast for a protein-rich meal with less saturated fat than red meat.
- **Plant-based protein sources:** Beans, lentils, tofu, and tempeh are good alternatives to animal protein, delivering important nutrients and fiber while containing less saturated fat.

Creating a Sustainable Heart-Healthy Diet

Making big dietary adjustments might be difficult. *Begin by making tiny, sustainable changes:*

- Replace sugary beverages with water or unsweetened tea.
- Include a dish of veggies with your lunch and dinner.
- Choose whole wheat bread over white bread.
- Reduce your portion amounts gradually.

Remember that consistency is crucial. By making tiny, lasting adjustments and concentrating on eating a range of nutritious foods, you can create a heart-healthy diet that will fuel your body and safeguard your cardiovascular health for years to come.

CHAPTER 9: UNSATURATED FATS: FRIENDS OR FOES?

In the world of nutrition, lipids are sometimes veiled in mystery, especially when it comes to heart health. This chapter distinguishes between healthy (unsaturated) and harmful (saturated and trans) fats, emphasizing their effects on the cardiovascular system and equipping you to make educated dietary choices.

The Fat Landscape

Fats are vital nutrients that perform several roles in the body, *including:*

- Energy Storage
- Hormone Production
- Cell Membrane Structure
- Absorption of fat-soluble vitamins (A, D, E, and K).

However, not all fats are created equally. Understanding the two major kinds of fats, saturated and unsaturated, and their effects on heart health is critical.

The antagonists: Saturated and trans fats

Saturated fats are largely found in animal products such as red meat, full-fat dairy, and processed meals.

Trans fats are mostly generated during the production of vegetable oils (partially hydrogenated oils) or occur naturally in tiny levels in red meat and dairy products.

Impact on heart health:

Saturated and trans fats raise LDL ("bad") cholesterol levels, causing plaque accumulation in arteries and raising the risk of a heart attack or stroke.

Reduce HDL ("good") cholesterol: These fats can also lower HDL cholesterol, which eliminates excess cholesterol from the bloodstream, endangering heart health.

Limit your consumption of saturated and trans fats. To lower your intake of these harmful fats, use lean protein sources, and low-fat dairy products, and avoid processed meals.

Protagonists: Unsaturated Fats

Monounsaturated fats are found in avocados, olive oil, nuts, and seeds.

Polyunsaturated fats can be found in fatty fish (such as salmon, tuna, and mackerel), flaxseeds, walnuts, and vegetable oils.

Impact on heart health:

Lower LDL ("bad") cholesterol: Unsaturated fats can help reduce LDL cholesterol, lowering the risk of plaque formation and heart disease.

Raise HDL ("good") cholesterol: These fats can also help to increase HDL cholesterol levels, which promotes heart health.

Additional benefits: Some unsaturated fats, notably omega-3 fatty acids found in fatty fish, may aid in reducing inflammation and improving blood pressure.

Accept unsaturated fats as part of a heart-healthy diet. Choose healthy cooking oils such as olive oil, include fatty fish in your meals, and eat nuts and seeds in moderation.

It's crucial to note that categorizing fats as "good" or "bad" is an oversimplified approach. While saturated and trans fats are typically harmful to heart health, some saturated fats found in plants, such as coconut oil, may have neutral or even favorable effects on cholesterol levels.

Finally, the most effective technique for promoting heart health is to eat a whole-food, balanced diet that is low in saturated and trans fats while including a modest quantity of unsaturated fats from a variety of sources.

Choosing Wisely

- Read the food labels: Pay attention to the kind and quantity of fat in packaged goods.
- Select lean cuts of beef and poultry.
- Choose low-fat or fat-free dairy products.
- Limit your intake of processed and fried meals, as well as baked items.
- Include healthy fats such as avocado, nuts, seeds, and olive oil in your diet.

Remember, while unsaturated fats are helpful to heart health, moderation is essential.

Understanding the significance of different types of fats and making educated decisions can help you make dietary adjustments that improve your heart and general health.

CHAPTER 10: THE SALT CONUNDRUM

Sodium, sometimes known as "salt," is a vital element that regulates fluid balance and transmits nerve signals. However, excessive salt consumption has been related to a major risk factor for heart disease: high blood pressure. This chapter delves into the dilemma of sodium, discussing its necessity, the hazards linked with overconsumption, and practical techniques for limiting salt intake for a healthier heart.

The Role of Sodium in the Body

Sodium serves various important functions in the body, *including*:

Maintaining fluid balance: Sodium regulates the quantity of fluid within and around cells, which contributes to normal blood volume and pressure.

Nerve impulse transmission: Sodium helps nerve signals travel throughout the body, providing correct muscle function and communication between the brain and other organs.

Sodium also aids in **muscular function**, digestion, and nutrition absorption.

How Too Much Salt Can Be Detrimental

While salt is necessary, excessive consumption can have serious repercussions, especially for blood pressure:

Impact on blood volume: When you take too much sodium, your body retains extra fluid to dilute the elevated sodium content in your blood. This increased fluid volume causes greater strain on your blood vessels, resulting in elevated blood pressure.

High blood pressure increases the chance of developing heart disease, stroke, and heart failure. Even little increases in blood pressure can greatly raise the risk of these illnesses.

Strategies for Salt Intake Moderation

The American Heart Association recommends that healthy persons restrict their salt consumption to less than 2,300 milligrams (mg) per day, and even lower (less than 1,500 mg/day) for those with high blood pressure or other health concerns. *Here are some techniques to help you manage your salt intake:*

Limit your intake of processed and restaurant foods, which are generally rich in added salt. Choose fresh, whole foods whenever feasible.

Read the food labels: Pay particular attention to the salt levels of each dish. When comparing similar items, choose those with lower salt concentrations.

Cooking more meals at home helps you to manage the quantity of salt used in your meals.

Use herbs and spices: Experiment with different herbs and spices to add flavor to your cuisine without using salt.

Gradually limit your salt consumption: Your taste senses will gradually acclimate to a decreased amount of salinity.

Seek expert assistance: If you're having trouble managing your salt consumption, talk to a registered dietitian or healthcare professional about individualized techniques.

Remember that eliminating all salt is not suggested. The key is moderation. By using the tactics indicated above and lobbying for reform in the food business, you may effectively traverse the salt environment, combining your basic requirements with heart health protection. This thoughtful approach enables

you to make more informed decisions, paving
the road for a healthy future.

CHAPTER 11: READING FOOD LABELS

In today's environment, traversing the grocery store aisle may be like decoding a hidden code. Food labels are dense with information, but interpreting them may be difficult. This chapter will teach you how to read labels and provide you with the knowledge and skills you need to make educated food choices that benefit your heart and general health.

Essential Components for Unlocking the Label

A food label generally has different crucial sections:

Serving size is important for determining how many of the nutrients and components mentioned apply to a single serving. Be wary of items with deceiving serving sizes; you may be consuming more than you know.

Calories: This represents the overall number of calories in each serving. While not the only measure of health, calorie intake must be matched with calorie expenditure to maintain a healthy weight.

Nutrients: This section lists the following nutrients:
Total fat, saturated fat, trans fat, and unsaturated fat. Pay attention to the kind and

amount of fat in your diet, focusing on unsaturated fats while reducing saturated and trans fats.

Cholesterol: Moderate consumption is typically suggested, with emphasis on dietary sources such as eggs and fatty fish over processed meals.

Sodium: Aim for reduced sodium levels to control blood pressure and preserve heart health.

Carbohydrates, fiber, and sugars: Choose whole grains and fiber-rich foods over processed carbs and added sweets.

Protein: Choose lean protein sources such as fish, chicken, beans, and almonds.

Ingredients are listed in descending order by weight. This helps you to identify the food's key components and evaluate their quality. Look for full, unprocessed foods at the top of the list, and avoid items with added sugars, bad fats, or artificial substances.

% Daily Value (%DV): This reflects how much of a given nutrient a single serving contributes to the recommended daily intake. It might be useful for comparing similar items and determining how a food fits into your overall nutritional requirements.

Tips for Effective Label Reading

Avoid "healthy" claims: Marketing phrases such as "healthy," "natural," and "low-fat" do not imply a healthy option. Always prioritize reading the nutritional facts.

Beware of hidden sugars: Added sugars can be disguised as "high-fructose corn syrup," "cane sugar," or "malt syrup."

Compare the products: When selecting similar things, check their nutritional composition to make educated choices.

Consider your nutritional demands and health objectives: Tailor your dietary selections to your specific requirements and health objectives, taking into mind any allergies or sensitivities you may have.

Do not rely exclusively on labels: Labels provide useful information, but they do not give the entire story. When making food choices, consider the overall quality and origin.

Learning to read food labels correctly gives you control over your dietary choices, which benefits your heart health and general well-being. Use the information presented in this chapter to confidently navigate the supermarket store, make informed judgments, and nourish your body with the finest potential options. Remember that consistency is crucial. By including label reading in your daily routine, you may develop the skills required to make educated decisions for a healthy future.

PART 4:

MOVING YOUR BODY – EXERCISE

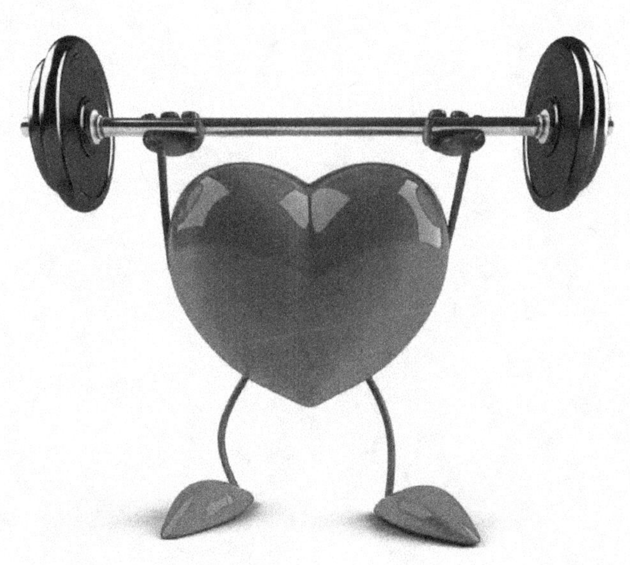

CHAPTER 12: FIND YOUR FIT

Physical activity is an essential component of a healthy lifestyle, promoting heart health and general well-being. However, the notion of exercising may often be intimidating, resulting in resistance and, ultimately, a lack of long-term participation. This chapter discusses the significance of choosing physical activities that you like, creating a long-term commitment to fitness that keeps you active and your heart healthy for years to come.

Benefits of Movement

Regular physical activity has far-reaching benefits beyond weight loss and appearance. *Here's how it helps your heart.*

Regular exercise strengthens the heart muscle, making it more effective in pumping blood throughout the body.

Lowers blood pressure: Physical exercise helps control blood pressure, which is a major risk factor for heart disease.

Exercise can help improve HDL ("good") cholesterol while decreasing LDL ("bad") cholesterol, therefore protecting your heart.

Reduces inflammation: Regular physical exercise helps to reduce chronic inflammation, which is a risk factor for a variety of health issues, including heart disease.

Boosts mood and decreases stress: Exercise produces endorphins, natural mood-enhancing chemicals, and aids in stress management, both of which are helpful to general well-being and can have an indirect influence on heart health.

Finding Activities You Love

Finding things that you truly like is crucial to making fitness a permanent habit.

Step outside of your comfort zone by trying new hobbies such as dance, swimming, hiking, rock climbing, or team sports.

Connect with others: Join a fitness class, locate a gym companion, or join in group activities to keep motivated and add some social interaction to your routine.

Focus on the fun: Prioritize activities that you love, rather than ones you believe you "should" participate in.

Celebrate minor successes: Recognize your accomplishments, no matter how minor, to stay motivated and celebrate your dedication to your well-being.

Listen to your body: Don't push yourself too hard, especially at first. To prevent injury and exhaustion, gradually increase the intensity and duration.

Incorporating Activity into Your Daily Life

Small modifications might have a major influence on your total exercise level.

- Take the stairs rather than the elevator.
- Park further from your location and walk.

- Perform bodyweight exercises or quick workouts during ad breaks.
- Incorporate exercise into your activities, such as biking, gardening, or dancing.
- Throughout the day, alternate between brief walks or stretches to avoid excessive sitting.

Tips for Building Sustainable Habits

Set realistic objectives: Begin with manageable goals and progressively raise the intensity and length of your exercise as you gain strength.

Find an accountability buddy: Having someone who supports and motivates you might help you remain on track.

Track your progress: To stay motivated, keep track of your activities and celebrate your accomplishments.

Be flexible and adaptive: Life occurs. Adjust your schedule as necessary to preserve consistency while accommodating unexpected events.

Reward Yourself: Celebrate your accomplishments with non-food rewards to foster good behavior.

Finding a workout regimen that you love is about appreciating the experience of movement rather than achieving a specific goal. By adding things you truly like and taking a long-term strategy, you may discover the joy of moving, protect your heart, and lay the groundwork for a healthier, happier you.

CHAPTER 13: THE MAGIC OF MODERATE EXERCISE

Physical activity might be difficult to prioritize in today's fast-paced society. However, the good news is that you don't have to devote hours to strenuous exercise to receive major heart health advantages. The secret is in moderate-intensity exercise, which provides several benefits for a healthy and happy heart. This chapter digs into the advantages of moderate-intensity exercise, provides examples to suit diverse tastes, and teaches you how to implement them into your everyday life.

Benefits of Moderate Exercise to your heart.

Regular moderate-intensity exercise has several benefits for your cardiovascular system:

Moderate-intensity exercise strengthens the heart muscle, causing it to work harder and pump blood more effectively throughout the body. This enhanced strength translates into better oxygen supply and waste disposal, which improves overall cardiovascular function.

Lowers blood pressure: Regular moderate exercise can help control blood pressure, which is a major risk factor for cardiovascular disease. Regular physical activity relaxes blood arteries and improves blood flow, which reduces strain on the heart.

Improves blood cholesterol levels: Moderate-intensity exercise can help balance cholesterol levels. It can help raise HDL ("good") cholesterol, which eliminates extra cholesterol from the bloodstream, and reduce LDL ("bad") cholesterol, lowering the risk of plaque accumulation in the arteries.

Aids in weight management: Regular physical exercise can help you maintain a healthy weight, which puts less strain on your heart and lowers your chance of developing numerous heart-related illnesses.

Increases mood and decreases stress: Moderate exercise causes the production of endorphins, which are natural mood-enhancing compounds that counteract stress hormones. This can enhance your general well-being while also indirectly contributing to heart health by reducing stress, which is a known risk factor for cardiovascular disease.

Examples of
moderate-intensity exercise.

The beauty of moderate-intensity exercise is its adaptability. *Here are some examples that are appropriate for different preferences:*

Brisk walking: This easily accessible workout may be done practically anywhere and requires no equipment. Aim for a speed that allows you to easily have a conversation.

Swimming: This low-impact sport is easy on your joints and provides a full-body workout. It is an excellent choice for people who have injuries or joint discomfort.

Riding: Whether done outdoors or on a stationary cycle, riding is a moderate-intensity activity that improves your legs and cardiovascular system.

Dancing: This enjoyable and sociable exercise increases your heart rate while activating your entire body. Explore a variety of genres, including Zumba, ballroom dancing, and simply dancing in your living room to your favorite music.

Gardening provides a moderate-intensity workout that includes bending, lifting, and walking.

Household chores: Even simple tasks such as brisk walking while cleaning, vacuuming, or mowing the lawn can count toward your daily moderate-intensity exercise goal.

Incorporating Moderate Exercise into Your Lifestyle

Incorporating and maintaining consistency is essential for obtaining the advantages of moderate-intensity exercise.

Begin small: Begin with brief bursts of moderate-intensity exercise, gradually increasing duration and frequency as your fitness improves.

Break it down: Aim for 150 minutes of moderate-intensity activity per week. You may divide this into 30-minute sessions five days a week, or shorter spurts throughout the day.

Find hobbies that you enjoy: Explore many possibilities to find things that you truly enjoy and find intriguing, making them simpler to persist with in the long run.

Incorporate movement into your daily routine: Look for ways to boost your daily activity level, such as using the stairs rather than the elevator, parking further away from your destination, or taking brief exercise breaks at work.

Listen to your body: Don't push yourself too hard, especially at the start. Pay heed to your body's cues and take rest days as needed to avoid injury and burnout.

Remember:

- Each step counts! Even tiny improvements in exercise can have a major impact on your heart health.
- Consistency is essential. For the best long-term results, aim for frequent moderate-intensity exercise.
- Consult your doctor before beginning any new workout regimen, especially if you have any underlying health concerns.

By including moderate-intensity exercise in your daily routine, you are not only moving your body but also taking control of your heart health and general well-being. Explore various activities, discover what speaks to you, and go on a path of exercise that is both pleasurable and helpful to your heart and life. The magic genuinely resides in its regularity and beneficial influence.

CHAPTER 14: STRENGTH IS KEY

While cardiovascular exercise is generally the focus of discussions about heart health, the importance of strength training is sometimes underestimated. This chapter discusses the advantages of adding strength training into your routine, emphasizing its influence on not just physical strength but also cardiovascular health and general well-being.

Benefits of Strength Training

Strength training, commonly referred to as resistance training, is the use of weights, body weights, or resistance bands to challenge and accelerate muscular growth. Contrary to common assumptions, it is not just about huge muscles. *Here are some of the surprising benefits it provides.*

Improved cardiovascular health: Strength training can help to enhance heart health in several ways. *It helps:*

- ***Strengthen the heart muscle:*** Strength training, like moderate-intensity exercise, helps the heart muscle pump blood more effectively throughout the body.

- ***Manage blood pressure:*** Regular strength exercise can help decrease blood pressure and lower the risk of heart disease.

- ***Improve blood sugar management:*** Strength training can boost insulin sensitivity, resulting in better blood sugar control and lowering the risk of type 2 diabetes, a risk factor for cardiovascular disease.

Maintain a healthy weight: Strength training improves and maintains muscle mass, which boosts metabolism and aids in weight control, eventually boosting heart health.

Strength training improves bone density, lowering the risk of osteoporosis, a disorder that weakens bones and raises the chance of fracture.

Strength training activities can enhance your balance and coordination, lowering your chance of falls and accidents, and so indirectly protect your heart health by averting problems.

Increased functional fitness: Strength training enhances your capacity to execute everyday tasks with ease, boosting your overall health and independence.

Improved mood and self-esteem: Seeing gains in strength and physical ability can lead to a more positive self-image and mood, which can have an indirect influence on general health.

Examples of Strength Training Exercises that Help You Build Your Arsenal

The beauty of strength training resides in its versatility.

Bodyweight exercises include using your body weight for **resistance**, such as squats, lunges, push-ups, planks, and dips.

Free weights: To target different muscle groups, execute workouts using dumbbells, barbells, or kettlebells.

Resistance bands are useful equipment that provide varying resistance levels and may be used for a variety of activities.

Weight machines: Gyms provide a variety of weight machines that may help you perform specialized workouts that target different muscle areas.

Including Strength Training in Your Routine

Here are some recommendations for safely and efficiently incorporating strength training into your regimen.

Begin with lesser weights or bodyweight exercises, then gradually increase the weight or intensity as you gain strength.

Focus on good form: To avoid injury, see a licensed personal trainer or utilize trusted resources to learn basic workout techniques.

Target all major muscle groups: Train all major muscle groups in your body at least twice a week, with adequate rest and recovery time in between sessions.

Listen to your body: Take rest days as needed and avoid overtraining and injuries.

Strength training is more than simply increasing muscle; it is an investment in your entire health. By adding yoga into your daily routine, you not only strengthen your body and improve your cardiovascular health, but you also increase your confidence, vitality, and functional capacity. Accept the challenge of strength training and see the good effects it has on your heart and life.

CHAPTER 15: OVERCOMING EXERCISE OBSTACLES FOR A HEALTHIER HEART

Adopting a better lifestyle via exercise might be difficult. This chapter provides you with practical solutions for overcoming typical exercise hurdles and maintaining consistency in your program, resulting in a healthier heart and a happier life.

Common exercise barriers and how to overcome them.

Several things might prevent us from beginning or keeping to an exercise plan. Recognizing these hurdles and finding tactics to overcome them is critical to success. *Here are some frequent issues and solutions:*

Lack of time:

Solution: Schedule your exercises ahead of time and regard them as crucial appointments. Use shorter, high-intensity exercises, or divide your activity into smaller, more manageable bits throughout the day.

Lack of motivation:

Solution: Engage in things you truly like. Set achievable objectives and appreciate your accomplishments, no matter how modest. Find a workout companion or join a group exercise class to boost motivation and accountability.

Fear of Failure:

Solution: Focus on making progress rather than achieving perfection. Do not compare yourself to others; everyone begins somewhere. Start slowly and progressively increase the intensity and duration of your exercises as you gain strength.

Intimidation at the gym:

Solution: Begin with home routines that incorporate bodyweight exercises or free weights. Consider alternatives such as outdoor activities, online fitness programs, or private workouts with a personal trainer.

Budget issues:

Solution: To address cost concerns, consider free or low-cost options such as bodyweight workouts, walking, running, and free internet resources. Consider purchasing basic fitness equipment such as resistance bands or a yoga mat for home training.

Physical limits or health issues:

Solution: Consult your doctor before beginning any new workout regimen, especially if you have any underlying health concerns. They can assist you in developing a safe and successful workout regimen that is tailored to your unique requirements and restrictions.

Maintaining consistency in your routine

Once you've passed the early barriers, the objective is to retain consistency.

Set SMART goals: Specific, Measurable, Attainable, Relevant, and Time-bound objectives give a clear path and a sense of success.

Find an accountability buddy: Share your objectives with a friend or family member, or join an online fitness community for motivation and support.

Track your progress: Track your workouts and praise your accomplishments. Seeing your success may be a tremendous incentive for staying on track.

Make it convenient: To avoid last-minute excuses, schedule your exercises at times that are convenient for you and prepare your training attire and equipment ahead of time.

Reward Yourself: Celebrate your accomplishments with non-food rewards to reinforce excellent behavior and keep you motivated.

Be flexible and adaptive: Life occurs. Adjust your schedule as necessary to preserve consistency while accommodating unexpected events.

Listen to your body: Don't push yourself too hard, especially at first. Take relaxation days and pay attention to your body's cues to avoid injuries and burnout.

Find delight in movement: Prioritize activities that you like over those that you believe you "should" perform. This makes exercise more sustainable and pleasurable in the long term.

Understanding and overcoming typical hurdles, as well as implementing the solutions provided in this chapter, can help you build a consistent workout regimen that matches your lifestyle and preferences. Remember that increasing your physical activity benefits your heart health, general well-being, and a happier, healthier future.

PART 5:

TAMING THE TIGER – STRESS MANAGEMENT

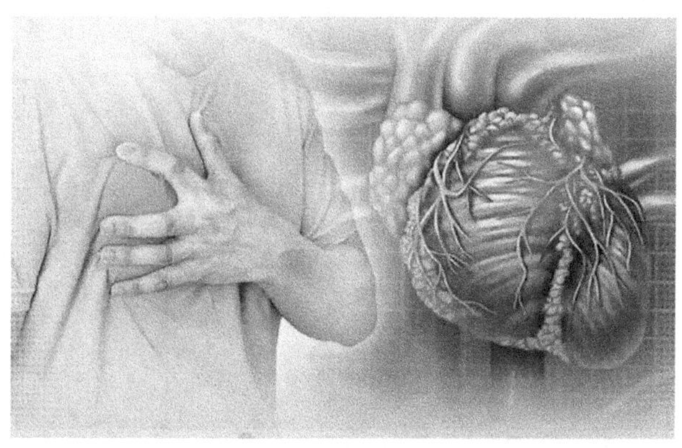

CHAPTER 16: THE HEART-STRESS CONNECTION

Stress is an unavoidable aspect of life. Chronic stress, defined as continuous periods of high tension and concern, can have a substantial influence on your health, particularly your heart. This chapter investigates the link between chronic stress and numerous heart disease risk factors, emphasizing the significance of stress management for a healthy heart.

Understanding Stress Response

When presented with a stressful scenario, your body activates the "fight-or-flight" reaction, a survival mechanism passed down from our ancestors. This reaction causes the production of chemicals such as adrenaline and cortisol, which:

Increase your heart rate and blood pressure: This will prepare your body for immediate action or escape.

Increase blood sugar levels to offer easily available energy.

Prioritize immediate survival by diverting resources away from other biological activities, such as digestion and immunological response.

While this reaction is critical in acute situations, chronic stress puts the body in a permanent state of fight-or-flight, *resulting in:*

Increased Risk Factors for Heart Disease

High blood pressure: Chronic activation of the stress response can result in persistently increased blood pressure, a major risk factor for cardiovascular disease.

Unhealthy blood cholesterol levels: Stress can cause changes in cholesterol levels, potentially increasing LDL ("bad") cholesterol while reducing HDL ("good") cholesterol, raising the risk of heart disease.

Inflammation: Chronic stress can cause low-grade inflammation throughout the body, weakening blood vessels and raising the risk of heart disease.

Blood clotting: Stress increases the risk of blood clots forming, which can block arteries and cause a heart attack or stroke.

Unhealthy lifestyle choices: Stress may lead to unhealthy habits such as smoking, binge eating, and physical inactivity, all of which raise the risk of heart disease.

The Effects of Stress on Mental and Emotional Wellbeing

Chronic stress can also have a substantial influence on your mental and emotional well-being, *perhaps causing:*

Anxiety and depression: These illnesses can worsen stress and harm your heart health.

Sleep disturbances: Sleep problems can hurt your overall health and raise your chance of developing heart disease.

Reduced stress tolerance: Chronic stress can make it more difficult to manage future stressful events, resulting in a vicious cycle.

Strategies for Effective Stress Management

Fortunately, some ways can help you manage stress and safeguard your heart health:

Identify and treat the source of stress: Understanding the underlying reason for your stress helps you to devise focused coping techniques.

Deep breathing, meditation, yoga, and gradual muscle relaxation are all useful approaches for reducing stress.

Engage in regular physical activity: Exercise is a great stress reliever and has various heart-health advantages.

Prioritize healthy sleep: Aim for 7-8 hours of excellent sleep every night to boost general well-being and stress reduction.

Maintain healthy dietary habits: Feed your body nourishing nutrients to maintain your physical and mental wellness during stressful times.

Connect with loved ones: Stress management relies heavily on social support. Surround yourself with positive, supporting individuals.

Seek professional help: If you're having trouble managing stress on your own, try seeing a therapist or counselor.

<u>*Remember:*</u>

- ***Chronic stress is not inevitable:*** Adopting appropriate stress management practices will help you safeguard your heart health and general well-being.

- ***Listen to your body and thoughts:*** Pay attention to your stress signals and treat them before they affect your health.

- ***Prioritize self-care:*** Engaging in enjoyable hobbies and self-care are vital for stress management and heart health.

Understanding the link between chronic stress and heart disease risk factors can empower you to take control of your health. Prioritizing stress management will help you live a better lifestyle for your heart, mind, and general well-being. Remember that every step toward stress reduction leads to a better and happier existence.

CHAPTER 17: IDENTIFYING STRESS TRIGGERS

Stress, like a thief in the night, may take your peace of mind and harm your health, especially your heart. This chapter teaches you how to identify your stress triggers, which are the conditions, ideas, or events that cause your fight-or-flight reaction. Recognizing your triggers allows you to handle them proactively, protecting your heart health and cultivating a more serene lifestyle.

Understanding Your Stress Response

When presented with a perceived threat, your body immediately activates the fight-or-flight reaction, a survival mechanism passed down from our ancestors. This response, defined by the production of chemicals such as adrenaline and cortisol, prepares you to face or flee the perceived threat. While this reaction is critical in emergencies, chronic activation due to prolonged stress can have a negative influence on your physical and emotional health, increasing your risk of heart disease.

The Triggers Lurk: Recognizing Stressors

Stress triggers are unique to each person. What causes stress for one individual may not impact another. The trick is to recognize your specific triggers. *Some stress triggers are:*

- **External variables** include job deadlines, hard workloads, and toxic office settings.
- Financial issues, debt, and employment uncertainty.
- Relationship issues, disputes, or a lack of support.
- Family issues, such as caring for aging parents or children.
- Health issues, personal ailments, or chronic diseases.
- Daily difficulties, traffic delays, lengthy commutes, and technical problems.

- **Internal causes** include negative self-talk, perfectionism, and excessive expectations.
- Fear of failure, public speaking anxiety, and social circumstances.

- Feeling overwhelmed, out of control, and unable to delegate.
- Saying no is difficult, as is accepting too much responsibility or setting bad limits.
- Feeling lonely, alone, or without social support.

Techniques for Identifying Your Triggers

When you are stressed, **practice mindfulness** by paying attention to your thoughts, feelings, and body sensations. Take note of the situations, events, or persons that have triggered these emotions.

Journaling: Record your actions, feelings, and any stressful occurrences that occur throughout the day. Over time, patterns may form that identify possible triggers.

Body awareness: Pay attention to bodily signs of stress, such as elevated heart rate, muscular tightness, headaches, or stomach distress. These commonly imply the presence of a trigger.

Identify the avoidance behaviors: When you're anxious, do you tend to retreat from social settings, procrastinate on work, or overeat? These actions can provide insights into underlying causes.

Seek external support: Consult with trustworthy friends, family members, or a therapist to gain objective perspectives and identify your triggers.

Know this:

- There is no one-size-fits-all answer. Your triggers are unique to you.

- ***Be honest with yourself;*** Recognize your triggers, no matter how trivial they may appear.

- ***The journey is continuous:*** Your triggers might change as you go through life. Regularly examine and change your stress management tactics.

Strategies to Manage Your Triggers Once Identified

Once you've identified your triggers, *you may proactively handle them through:*

Avoidance: Avoid circumstances that routinely elicit your stress reaction.

Preparation: If avoidance is not an option, prepare yourself for the scenario. Develop coping strategies such as deep breathing exercises and positive self-talk.

Communication: Be open about your wants and limits with people to reduce stress triggers in your interactions.

Time management: Prioritize activities, delegate when feasible, and set realistic deadlines to prevent being overwhelmed.

Relaxation Techniques: To cope with stress at the moment, practice relaxation techniques such as deep breathing, meditation, or yoga regularly.

Seek professional help: If you are unable to handle your stress on your own, you might consider seeing a therapist or counselor.

Identifying your stressors is the first step toward a more relaxed and healthy existence. By learning to recognize and control them, you can protect your heart health, enhance your general well-being, and create a feeling of calm and resilience in the face of life's difficulties. Remember that you are not alone on this road, and by taking control of your stress reaction, you are enabling yourself to flourish.

CHAPTER 18: RELAXATION TECHNIQUES FOR EVERY LIFESTYLE

In today's fast-paced society, stress has become a common occurrence. Chronic stress, on the other hand, can have a negative influence on both your physical and mental health, increasing your chance of developing heart disease. This chapter exposes you to several relaxation techniques designed to fit diverse lives and interests. By implementing these techniques into your everyday routine, you may achieve inner peace, efficiently manage stress, and protect your heart health.

Understanding the power of relaxation

Relaxation methods are an effective stress-reduction strategy. *They activate your body's relaxing response by:*

- Lowering your heart rate and blood pressure.
- Slowing down your breathing rate.
- Reducing muscular tension.
- Calming the mind and improving sleep quality.
- Increasing general well-being.

The appeal of these strategies rests in their versatility and accessibility. Whether you have five minutes or an hour, there is a relaxing technique to suit your hectic schedule and individual tastes.

A Spectrum of Relaxation Techniques.

Mindfulness is the discipline of concentrating one's attention on the present moment without judgment. Activities such as mindful walking, mindful eating, and just noticing your breath can help you develop present-moment awareness and reduce stress.

Meditation is a discipline that trains your focus and awareness. Transcendental Meditation, Mindfulness Meditation, and Guided Meditation are three diverse meditation practices that each provide a unique approach to obtaining inner tranquility.

Deep Breathing: This basic yet effective approach comprises slow, regulated breathing exercises. Techniques such as diaphragmatic breathing increase your body's relaxation response, which promotes peace and reduces tension.

Progressive Muscle Calm: This technique includes gradually tensing and releasing various muscle groups throughout your body, which promotes both physical and mental calm.

Yoga is an ancient discipline that incorporates physical postures, breathing exercises, and meditation. Different yoga styles, ranging from moderate Hatha yoga to more strenuous Vinyasa yoga, cater to a variety of fitness levels and interests, providing a comprehensive approach to stress relief.

Visualization is a technique for forming mental pictures of serene sights or experiences. By using your imagination, you can trigger the relaxation response and reduce tension.

Tai Chi is a peaceful workout that includes slow, flowing motions, deep breathing, and meditation. Tai Chi promotes relaxation, increases balance and flexibility, and lowers stress.

Listening to Calming Music: Relaxing music may have a significant impact on your mood and stress level. Choose music with slow tempos and soothing melodies to help you relax and sleep better.

Selecting Techniques That Resonate With You

Experiment: Try different relaxation techniques to see what works for you.

Start small: Begin with short workouts and progressively increase the time as you gain confidence.

Stay consistent: Regular practice is essential for realizing the long-term advantages of relaxation methods.

Create a calm setting: Find a peaceful, distraction-free location and create a relaxing atmosphere.

Be patient: Learning a new relaxation method requires time and practice. Be patient with yourself, and enjoy the process.

Incorporating relaxation techniques into your daily routine not only helps you manage stress but also benefits your entire health and well-being. The approaches discussed in this chapter provide a variety of possibilities, allowing you to discover what works best for you and build a sense of inner calm. Remember, a calmer self leads to a healthier heart, laying the groundwork for a happier and more fulfilled life.

CHAPTER 19: BUILDING RESILIENCE

Life is an unavoidable journey full of both pleasures and difficulties. While stress is a normal reaction to life's challenges, prolonged stress can have a negative influence on both physical and mental health, raising the risk of heart disease. This chapter looks into the notion of emotional resilience and provides practical ways for developing inner strength so that you may handle stress and traverse life's obstacles more easily.

Understanding Emotional Resilience

Emotional resilience refers to the ability to adapt and recover from difficult events, disappointments, and adversity. *The inner strength enables you to:*

- Handle life's ups and downs without becoming overwhelmed.
- Maintain an optimistic attitude, even in adverse conditions.
- Challenges and failures serve as opportunities for growth.
- Recover from hardship with increased strength and perspective.

Developing emotional resilience is critical for managing stress and protecting your heart health. By developing your inner strength, you can better deal with life's inevitable challenges, lessening their detrimental influence on your physical and emotional health.

The Pillars of Resilience

Here are several crucial aspects which helps to promote emotional resilience:

Acceptance: Embracing truth, especially when it is painful, permits you to go forward more clearly.

Maintaining a cheerful and optimistic attitude promotes hope and motivation throughout difficult circumstances.

Self-awareness: Understanding your thoughts, feelings, and reactions allows you to respond to events deliberately and efficiently.

Strong problem-solving abilities enable you to approach difficulties proactively and identify answers.

Emotional regulation: Learning to successfully regulate your emotions might help you avoid feeling overwhelmed in difficult situations.

Social support: Having a strong network of friends, family, or a therapist may give vital coping tools and a sense of belonging.

Meaning and purpose: Understanding your life's purpose and direction may bring inspiration and fortitude throughout difficult times.

Practical Strategies for Increasing Inner Strength

Mindfulness activities help you become more aware of your thoughts and emotions while remaining judgment-free, fostering emotional control and acceptance.

Challenge negative thought habits: Identify and counter negative self-talk that can worsen stress and reduce resilience.

Develop good coping techniques: Exercise, relaxation methods, and spending time in nature are all things that can help you manage stress more successfully.

Connect with others: Develop and maintain healthy relationships with people who may give encouragement and empathy during difficult times.

Seek professional help: If you are having difficulty managing stress or building resilience on your own, you might consider consulting with a therapist or counselor.

Celebrate your successes: Recognize and appreciate your development and accomplishments, no matter how minor, to increase your confidence and resilience.

Learn from your experiences: View adversities as chances for learning and growth, which will help you emerge stronger and more resilient.

Developing emotional resilience not only builds inner strength but also invests in a healthier heart and a more happy life. The tactics presented in this chapter can help you become a more resilient person, capable of navigating life's problems with greater ease, successfully managing stress, and cultivating a feeling of calm and well-being in the face of life's inevitable ups and downs. Remember that your path to resilience begins with a single step, and every effort counts toward increasing your inner strength and protecting your heart health.

CONCLUSION

As we approach the conclusion of *"Vitality Blueprint: Your Roadmap to a Heart-Healthy Life,"* we find ourselves at a crossroads between information and action. This book has shown a comprehensive strategy for avoiding heart disease, highlighting the complex link between lifestyle choices and cardiovascular health. Remember, the blueprint you've received is yours to personalize and use on your path to a bright and healthy life.

Key takeaways:

Adopt a holistic approach: Nurturing all elements of your life will help your heart thrive. This involves eating a well-balanced diet, getting regular exercise, successfully managing stress, and emphasizing self-care.

Navigate the Nutritional Landscape: Discover the benefits of a heart-healthy diet high in fruits and vegetables, whole grains, and lean protein. Learn to read food labels, make educated decisions, and enjoy a variety of nutritious and tasty meals.

Embrace movement and exercise: Physical activity, from moderate-intensity cardio to strength training, is essential for heart health. Find activities you like, incorporate them into your daily routine, and celebrate your accomplishments.

Overcome fitness barriers: Don't let common roadblocks like a lack of time, motivation, or intimidation derail your development. Find innovative ideas, create achievable objectives, and enjoy moving because every step counts.

Master the art of stress management: Chronic stress can have a negative influence on your cardiovascular health. Mindfulness, relaxation exercises, and self-care activities are powerful approaches for cultivating inner calm and resilience.

Empower Your Heart-Healthy Journey:

You're not alone on this journey. *Below are some information and tools to help you:*

Consult your doctor: Before beginning any new fitness regimen or making any nutritional changes, especially if you have any underlying health concerns, obtain customized advice from your physician.

Use resources: Investigate internet resources, trustworthy health information websites, and instructional materials from credible organizations such as the American Heart Association and the Centers for Disease Control and Prevention.

Connect with others: Join a support group, find a gym companion, or interact with health and wellness-focused online groups. Sharing your experience with others helps increase motivation and accountability.

Celebrate your progress: Recognize and appreciate your accomplishments, no matter how large or small, to stay encouraged and keep moving forward. Track your progress and reward yourself as you hit milestones.

Maintaining a healthy heart is a lifetime commitment. The "Vitality Blueprint" has provided you with the information and resources necessary to go on this journey. By using the skills you've learned, you can empower yourself to take charge of your health, handle stress efficiently, and lay the groundwork for a successful and heart-healthy future. Remember that each activity, each step toward a healthy lifestyle, has a big impact on your overall health. So, enjoy the trip, find delight in good habits, and invest in the health of your heart, which is the foundation of your vitality and happiness.

Remember, this is only the beginning. Put everything you've learned into action to maximize the potential of your "Vitality Blueprint" for a better and happier existence!

Dear Readers,

Thank you for joining me on this road to a heart-healthy lifestyle with "Vitality Blueprint." I hope the knowledge and techniques you discovered inspired you to pursue a path to improved well-being.

As I work to further develop the "Vitality Blueprint," your feedback is invaluable. Sharing your ideas and experiences will help me keep this book as a helpful resource for people like you, encouraging them to take charge of their health and lead satisfying lives.

Here's how you can help:

Leave a review: Provide honest comments. Your review can help prospective readers find this resource and make educated choices about their health journeys.

Spread the word! Share your "Vitality Blueprint" experience with friends, family, and health and wellness-related online groups. By increasing awareness about the benefits of a healthy lifestyle, you may inspire others to discover their own "Vitality Blueprint."

By sharing your views and experiences, you help shape the future of "Vitality Blueprint" and inspire others to begin on their paths to vibrant health and a joyful heart.

Thank you for taking part in this trip.

Sincerely,
Mercy Eunice